BEATING GOUT NATURALLY

The Truth About Gout's Causes, Signs, Symptoms, Prevention, And The Best Natural Treatments & Solutions For Ending Gout Pain Permanently!

DR. EDWARD THOMAS

Copyright © 2020

All rights reserved.

ISBN: 9798615909122

TEXT COPYRIGHT © [DR. EDWARD THOMAS]

all rights reserved. No part of this guide may be reproduced in any form without permission in writing from the publisher except in the case of brief quotations embodied in critical articles or reviews.

Legal & disclaimer

The information contained in this book and its contents is not designed to replace or take the place of any form of medical or professional advice; and is not meant to replace the need for independent medical, financial, legal or other professional advice or services, as may be required. The content and information in this book have been provided for educational and entertainment purposes only.

The content and information contained in this book have been compiled from sources deemed reliable, and it is accurate to the best of the author's knowledge, information, and belief. However, the author cannot guarantee its accuracy and validity and cannot be held liable for any errors and/or omissions. Further, changes are periodically made to this book as and when needed. Where appropriate and/or necessary, you must consult a professional (including but not limited to your doctor, attorney, financial advisor or such other professional advisor) before using any of the suggested remedies, techniques, or information in this book.

Upon using the contents and information contained in this book, you agree to hold harmless the author from and against any damages, costs, and expenses, including any legal fees potentially resulting from the application of any of the information provided by this book. This disclaimer applies to any loss, damages or injury caused by the use and application, whether directly or indirectly, of any advice or information presented, whether for breach of contract, tort, negligence, personal injury, criminal intent, or under any other cause of action.

You agree to accept all risks of using the information presented inside this book.

You agree that by continuing to read this book, where appropriate and/or necessary, you shall consult a professional (including but not limited to your doctor, attorney, or financial advisor or such other advisor as needed) before using any of the suggested remedies, techniques, or information in this book.

Table of Contents

INTRODUCTION 5

WHAT IS GOUT? 6

GOUT SYMPTOMS 8

GOUT CAUSES 10

WHAT CAN TRIGGER A GOUT ATTACK? 12

GOUT DIAGNOSIS 13

GOUT TREATMENTS 15

TIPS FOR MANAGING AN ATTACK AT HOME 17

TREATMENTS TO PREVENT GOUT ATTACKS 18

NATURAL REMEDIES FOR GOUT 24

A GOUT-FRIENDLY MENU FOR ONE WEEK 33

OTHER TIPS FOR REDUCING GOUT FLARE-UPS 35

THE GOUT DIET 36

THE BOTTOM LINE 38

CONCLUSION 39

CHECK OUT OTHER BOOKS 41

INTRODUCTION

The best and most concise resource for diagnosis and treatment of gout!

Gout is increasing in incidence, all over the world. In many countries, gout has become the leading cause of death. However, recent research has shown that up to 78% of doctors do not treat gout properly. Needless to say, there is a great need for more rapid advancements in diagnosis and treatment of this devastating disease.

If you or a loved one has gout and want to understand more about how gout starts and spreads and natural gout treatment, then this book is for you.

This is one of the most comprehensive books available on alternative treatments for gout.

This book contains proven steps and strategies on how to prevent, treat and fight gout permanently. It explains the treatments used successfully by a health professional/gout survivor of 30 years and by some of the leading medical and health practitioners currently in the field. This book is also for you if you are a high school or college student taking biology or a related topic and want to learn more about gout. This book is also a useful introduction to gout biology for medical students and PhD students, although it might be considered a bit basic by some students at that level.

I hope you enjoy your reading.

Let's get started!

WHAT IS GOUT?

Gout is a type of arthritis that causes pain similar to osteoarthritis, though there are some distinct differences.

It's caused by high uric acid buildup in the blood. Uric acid then accumulates in joints, causing inflammation with discomfort and pain. It's more common in men and you're more likely to get it as you get older.

TYPES OF GOUT

There are various stages through which gout progresses, and these are sometimes referred to as different types of gout.

Asymptomatic hyperuricemia

It is possible for a person to have elevated uric acid levels without any outward symptoms. At this stage, treatment is not required, though urate crystals may deposit in tissue and cause slight damage.

People with asymptomatic hyperuricemia may be advised to take steps to address any possible factors contributing to uric acid build-up.

Acute gout

This stage occurs when the urate crystals that have been deposited suddenly cause acute inflammation and intense pain. This sudden attack is referred to as a "flare" and will normally subside within 3 to 10 days. Flares can sometimes be triggered by stressful events, alcohol and drugs, as well as cold weather.

Interval or intercritical gout

This stage is the period in between attacks of acute gout. Subsequent flares may not occur for months or years, though if not treated, over time, they can last longer and occur more frequently. During this interval, further urate crystals are being deposited in tissue.

Chronic tophaceous gout

Chronic tophaceous gout is the most debilitating type of gout. Permanent damage may have occurred in the joints and the kidneys. The patient can suffer from chronic arthritis and develop tophi, big lumps of urate crystals, in cooler areas of the body such as the joints of the fingers.

It takes a long time without treatment to reach the stage of chronic tophaceous gout - around 10 years. It is very unlikely that a patient receiving proper treatment would progress to this stage.

Pseudogout

One condition that is easily confused with gout is pseudogout. The symptoms of pseudogout are very similar to those of gout, although thr flare-ups are usually less severe.

The major difference between gout and pseudogout is that the joints are irritated by calcium pyrophosphate crystals rather than urate crystals. Pseudogout requires different treatment to gout.

GOUT SYMPTOMS

Attacks

When you have gout, urate crystals can build up in your joints for years without you knowing they are there. When there are a lot of crystals in your joints, some of them can spill out from the cartilage into the space between the two bones in a joint.

The tiny, hard, sharp crystals can rub against the soft lining of the joint, called the synovium, causing a lot of pain swelling and inflammation. When this happens, it's known as an attack or flare of gout.

During an attack of gout the affected joint becomes:

- very painful
- tender
- red
- hot
- swollen.

The skin over the joint often appears shiny and may peel off a little as the attack settles.

Attacks usually come on very quickly, often during the night. Doctors describe this sudden development of symptoms as 'acute'.

The attack usually settles after about five to seven days, but it can go on for longer.

If gout is left untreated, attacks can become more common and may spread to new joints.

Attacks typically affect the joint at the base of the big toe and often start in the early hours of the morning. The symptoms develop quickly and are at their worst within just 12 to 24 hours of first noticing that anything is wrong.

Any light contact with the affected joint is very painful – even the weight of a bedsheet or wearing a sock can be unbearable.

Although gout most often affects the big toe, other joints may also be affected, including:

- other joints in your feet
- ankles
- knees
- elbows
- wrists
- fingers.

It's possible for several joints to be affected at the same time. It's not common to have gout in joints towards the centre of your body, such as the spine, shoulders or hips.

Gout attacks are especially common in joints at the ends of your legs and arms, such as in your fingers and toes. This is probably because these parts of the body are cooler, and low temperatures make it more likely for crystals to form.

Similar attacks can be caused by a condition called acute calcium pyrophosphate crystal arthritis. This is also known as acute CPP crystal arthritis, which used to be called 'pseudogout'.

Tophi

Urate crystals can also collect outside of the joints and can be seen under the skin, forming small, firm lumps called tophi. You can sometimes see the white colour of the urate crystals under the skin.

The most common areas for tophi are:

- over the top of the toes
- back of the heel
- front of the knee
- backs of the fingers and wrists
- around the elbow
- the ears.

Tophi aren't usually painful, but they can get in the way of normal daily activities. They can sometimes become inflamed, break down and leak pus-like fluid with gritty white material - these are the urate crystals.

Tophi can also grow within your joints and cause damage to your cartilage and bone. This can lead to more regular, daily pain when you use the affected joints.

GOUT CAUSES

There are two different types of gout. When you have it and there's no single cause, it's called primary gout. When you have it and it's caused by something else, it's known as secondary gout. Secondary gout can be caused by either:

- chronic kidney disease
- long-term use of medications that affect how well your kidneys can remove urate from your body.

RISK FACTORS

Family history

Even though your kidneys can be completely healthy, sometimes the genes you've inherited make it more likely that your kidneys don't flush urate out as well as they should. This is the most common cause of primary gout, especially when several family members are affected, such as your parents or grandparents.

Being overweight

Gout is much more common in people who are overweight. The more overweight you are, the more urate your body produces, and this may be more than your kidneys can cope with.

Being overweight also makes it more likely that you'll have:

- high blood pressure
- type 2 diabetes
- high cholesterol
- fats in your blood.

These conditions can all lower how much urate is filtered out by your kidneys.

Gender and age

Gout is about four times more common in men than women. It can affect men of any age, but the risk is greater as you get older.

Women rarely develop gout before the menopause. This is because the female hormone oestrogen increases how much urate is filtered out by the kidneys. But after the menopause, oestrogen levels go down and urate levels go up.

Taking certain medications

Some medications can reduce your kidneys' ability to get rid of urate properly. These include diuretics, also known as water tablets, and several tablets for high blood pressure, including beta-blockers and ACE inhibitors.

Other conditions

Several different conditions are linked to raised urate levels. This could be because they affect the way the kidneys filter urate, or because they cause more urate to be produced in the first place.

For some conditions, the link with gout is less clear, and may be due to many different factors.

Common conditions associated with gout include:

- chronic kidney disease
- high cholesterol and fats in the blood
- high blood pressure
- type 2 diabetes
- osteoarthritis.

WHAT CAN TRIGGER A GOUT ATTACK?

Several things can cause the crystals to shake loose into your joint cavity, triggering an attack. These include:

- a knock or injury to the joint
- an illness that may make you feverish
- having an operation
- having an unusually large meal, especially a fatty meal
- drinking too much alcohol
- dehydration
- starting urate lowering therapy, especially at a high dose, or not taking your treatment regularly each day.

GOUT DIAGNOSIS

Diagnosing gout is usually straightforward, especially if you have typical symptoms of the condition - for example, if you have an attack in your big toe.

But gout can sometimes be more difficult to diagnose. Your doctor will need to know about the symptoms you've been having and will probably need to perform some tests.

Blood tests

Blood tests to measure your urate levels can be helpful to support a diagnosis of gout, but aren't enough on their own to confirm it.

High urate levels in blood tests can suggest that you have gout, but this will need to be considered alongside your symptoms. It's possible to have high levels of urate, but not have any other symptoms of the condition.

Imaging tests

Ultrasound and CT scans can be good at spotting joint damage, crystals in the joints and early signs of gout. X-rays are generally used to pick up the bone and joint damage caused by having gout for a long time.

Synovial fluid examinations

These are a good way to rule out other crystal conditions and make a diagnosis.

They're done by taking a sample of your synovial fluid through a needle inserted into one of your joints. The fluid is then examined under a microscope for urate crystals. If you have tophi, doctors can take a sample from one of those instead.

How will gout affect me?

Attacks can vary from person to person. Some people only have an attack every few years, while others have attacks every few months.

Without medication attacks tend to happen more often and other joints can become affected.

Having high urate levels and gout for a long time can lead to other health problems, including:

- narrowing of the arteries - which can lead to an increased risk of stroke or heart attacks or other heart problems
- osteoarthritis, which occurs when the urate crystals and hard tophi cause joint damage.
- an increased risk of developing kidney disease or worsening of the condition if you already have it
- kidney stones
- an increased risk of some cancers, especially prostate cancer
- mental health problems, including depression
- underactive thyroid
- erectile dysfunction in men.

If you take medication to lower your urate levels, and have a healthy diet and lifestyle, most of the damage and complications caused by gout can be stopped.

GOUT TREATMENTS

Treatments for gout are incredibly successful. There are two main parts to treating gout, which are:

- treating the acute attack
- treatments to prevent future attacks.

Treating a gout attack

Treating an attack of gout doesn't lower your urate levels or stop future attacks. The treatment helps you to manage your symptoms when an attack happens.

The most commonly used drug treatments for attacks of gout are:

- non-steroidal anti-inflammatory drugs (NSAIDs)
- colchicine
- steroids.

Some people will be better suited to NSAIDS, while others will be suited to colchicine. But your preference is also taken into consideration – many people with gout quickly learn what works best for them.

In cases where one drug doesn't seem to be working on its own, your doctor might suggest a combination of NSAIDs with either colchicine or steroids.

Non-steroidal anti-inflammatory drugs (NSAIDs)

Attacks of gout are often treated with NSAID tablets, which can help with pain and reduce some of your inflammation. Ibuprofen, Naproxen and diclofenac are three NSAIDs you could be given.

If you've been prescribed NSAIDs to treat an attack, you should start taking them as soon as you notice signs of one coming on. Your doctor may let you keep a supply so you can start taking them at the first signs of an attack.

The earlier you start treatment, the better.

NSAIDs aren't suitable for everyone, so talk to your doctor about them first if you have any other conditions. They can also interact with other drugs, so make sure you talk to a doctor before starting on any new medication.

NSAIDs aren't usually prescribed for a long period of time, as they can cause problems with your digestive system. To reduce the risk of this happening and to protect your stomach, your doctor will also prescribe a proton pump inhibitor.

Colchicine

Colchicine isn't a painkiller, but can be very effective at reducing the inflammation caused by urate crystals.

As with NSAIDs, colchicine tablets should be taken as soon as you notice an attack coming on, or it may not work as well. Your doctor will probably recommend keeping a supply at home.

Colchicine can interact with several other drugs, including statins taken for high cholesterol. Your doctor will advise whether you'd be better off using an NSAID instead, or adjusting your other medications while you're taking colchicine.

You should avoid taking colchicine if you have chronic kidney disease.

Colchicine tablets can cause diarrhoea or stomach aches.

Steroids

If colchicine or NSAIDs haven't worked for you, or if you're at risk of side effects from these drugs, your doctor may prescribe steroids.

They are usually taken as a short course of tablets, lasting a few days.

However, they can also be taken as an injection into a muscle or joint affected by gout. This can be particularly helpful if gout is affecting only one joint.

Check out our steroids and steroid injection pages for more information.

TIPS FOR MANAGING AN ATTACK AT HOME

- Keep the area cool – an ice pack, or a bag of frozen peas wrapped in a tea towel, can be particularly good at reducing some of the pain and swelling.
- Rest the affected joint.
- Think about getting yourself a bed cage. These support the bedsheets above your feet so that your affected joint can rest without the strain of the sheets.

TREATMENTS TO PREVENT GOUT ATTACKS

There are drugs available that can lower urate levels, prevent new crystals from forming and dissolve away the crystals in your joints. They are called urate lowering therapies or ULTs for short.

Treatment with ULTs is generally started after an attack of gout has completely gone.

There's no single fixed dose of a ULT, and different people need different doses to get to the right blood urate level.

It can take a few months or years for the drugs to completely clear your body of urate crystals. But once they're gone, you will no longer have attacks of gout, tophi or risk of joint damage due to gout.

It's important to remember that ULTs won't stop attacks of gout straight away. You could actually have more attacks within the first six months of starting them.

Don't stop taking your ULTs if this happens to you, as this is actually a sign that the drugs are working. As the drugs start dissolving the crystals, they become smaller and are more likely to get into the joint cavity, triggering an attack.

Your doctor might suggest taking a low dose of colchicine or NSAID as a precaution against attacks during the first six months of starting ULTs.

ULTs are usually life-long treatments and require yearly check-ups to monitor your urate levels. If your symptoms aren't getting under control, talk to your doctor about your urate level, as you might need to be on a higher dose.

Try not to miss or skip any of your doses, especially in the first year or two of starting treatment. This could cause your urate levels to go up and down, which could trigger an attack.

Allopurinol

Allopurinol is the most commonly used ULT. It's a very effective treatment for most people with gout.

It works by reducing the amount of urate that your body makes.

You'll start on a low dose of allopurinol, which can be gradually increased until you are on the right dose.

Gradually building up the dose means it's less likely to trigger an attack and also makes sure you'll have the lowest dose needed to get your gout under control.

Allopurinol is broken down and removed from the body through your kidneys, so if you have a problem with your kidneys, it may not be suitable for you. Your doctor might decide to start you on an even lower dose and increase slowly, or suggest that you try febuxostat instead.

Febuxostat

Febuxostat is a newer drug that reduces the amount of urate made in the body in the same way that allopurinol does.

You won't be prescribed febuxostat as your first ULT, unless your doctor has said that you can't take allopurinol.

It works in a similar way to allopurinol but, instead of being broken down by the kidneys, it's broken down by your liver. It's useful if you have kidney problems and can't take a high enough dose of allopurinol.

Febuxostat is more likely to trigger gout attacks than allopurinol when you first start treatment. So, as a precaution, it's likely you'll be prescribed a low-dose NSAID or colchicine to take on a daily basis for the first six months of starting febuxostat.

There are just two doses of febuxostat, so if your urate levels haven't lowered enough after a month on the low dose, you may need to go on to the higher dose.

Uricosuric drugs

Uricosuric drugs, which include sulfinpyrazone, benzbromarone and probenecid, work by flushing out more urate than normal through your kidneys.

They're not used much in the UK, as they're not widely available. They'll only be prescribed by a rheumatologist if allopurinol and febuxostat haven't worked or aren't suitable for you.

It's unlikely you'll be able to take these drugs if you've had severe problems with your kidneys or had kidney stones. This is because, by encouraging your kidneys to filter more urate, they also increase the risk of developing kidney stones.

Uricosuric drugs are usually used on their own. But in rare cases, where you've tried several ULTs and none have worked for you, uricosurics can be used in combination with other ULTs, like allopurinol or febuxostat.

If you're unable to take allopurinol, febuxostat or a uricosuric, or if they don't work for you, you'll need to see a rheumatologist for advice.

Treatment for joint damage

If your gout has caused damage to your joints, then the treatments available will be the same as those used for osteoarthritis. They include:

- exercising regularly
- reducing the strain on your affected joints
- staying at a healthy weight
- taking painkillers
- in more severe cases, joint replacement surgery.

Managing your symptoms

Lifestyle choices are not the main reason why most people get gout.

However, if you have a healthy lifestyle and also take prescribed medication, you'll have the best chance of lowering your urate levels. This will then decrease the chances of you having attacks of gout.

Exercise

Exercise is extremely important, not only to reduce the chances of an attack, but also for your general health and wellbeing.

It doesn't matter how much exercise you do - a little is better than none at all.

Start off slowly and gradually build up how much you do until you're doing regular sessions.

As your confidence increases, you can increase the length and intensity of what you're doing.

Exercises that get you out of breath are particularly good for burning calories. You could try dancing, walking in hilly countryside or doubles tennis.

It helps to find a sport or exercise you enjoy which you enjoy and will keep doing. Some people find joining a leisure centre or sports club to be really fun and motivational. Have a look around and see what's available in your area.

You should avoid exercising during a flare up of gout, as it could make your pain worse. It's important to rest and recover and begin exercising after the pain and swelling has gone down.

Diet

You should try to have a well-balanced diet that is low in fats and added sugars, but high in vegetables and fibre.

Extreme weight loss or starvation diets increase cell breakdown in your body, which can raise urate levels. However, you should be OK to do some daytime fasting - for example, during Ramadan.

We don't recommend Atkins-type weight-loss diets, as they include a lot of meat and are high in purines.

If you're overweight, weight loss should be gradual combined with daily exercise.

The NHS has a good diet and exercise plan which can help you lose weight in a healthy way over 12 weeks.

Food to have in moderation

You should try to avoid eating large quantities of foods that are high in purines. But there's no need to remove them completely from your diet.

These include:

- red meat, game and offal - such as venison, kidneys, rabbit and liver
- seafood, particularly oily fish and shellfish - such as anchovies, fish roe, herring, mussels, crab and sardines
- foods rich in yeast extracts - such as Marmite, Bovril and Vegemite
- processed foods and drinks.

Protein is an important part of your diet, but you can get it from sources other than just meat and fish. You could try replacing a portion of meat with other protein-rich foods like soybeans, eggs, pulses or dairy products.

The UK Gout Society has a detailed food list of foods high in purines. Check out their diet factsheet for more information.

What about drink?

If you have gout and a history of kidney stones, you should try to drink at least two litres of water a day to decrease the chance of stones forming.

Sweetened soft drinks should be avoided, as they contain large amounts of sugar and can increase the risk of getting gout.

While fruit and fresh fruit juices contain sugar, the benefits of eating fruit are likely to far outweigh any negatives. Reducing how much sugar you consume from other sources is a heathier option than cutting out some of your five a day.

Alcohol

Drinking too much alcohol, especially beer and spirits, can increase your urate levels and your chances of triggering a gout attack. Beer is particularly bad, as it contains a lot of purines.

However, drinking a bit of wine doesn't appear to increase the risk of triggering an attack.

As a rule of thumb, try to stick to the government guidelines of drinking no more than 14 units a week. This is equivalent to about 6 pints of beer or 6 glasses of wine. But don't save these units up and drink them all in one go - it's better to spread them out over the course of the week.

Your doctor might also advise a lower limit.

NATURAL REMEDIES FOR GOUT

Cherries or tart cherry juice

According to a 2016 survey, cherries - whether sour, sweet, red, black, in extract form, as a juice, or raw - are a very popular and potentially successful home remedy for many.

One 2012 study and another that same year also suggest cherries may work to prevent gout attacks.

This research recommends three servings of any cherry form over a two-day period, which was considered the most effective.

Magnesium

Magnesium is a dietary mineral. Some claim it's good for gout because deficiency of magnesium may worsen chronic inflammatory stress in the body, though no studies prove this.

Still, a 2015 study showed that adequate magnesium is associated with lower and healthier levels of uric acid, thus potentially lowering gout risk. This applied to men but not women within the study.

Try taking magnesium supplements, but read label directions closely. Or, eat magnesium-rich foods daily. This may decrease gout risk or gout occurrence long term.

Ginger

Ginger is a culinary food and herb prescribed for inflammatory conditions. Its ability to help gout is well-documented.

One study found topical ginger reduced pain related to uric acid in gout. Another study showed that in subjects with high levels of uric acid (hyperuricemia), their serum uric acid level was reduced by ginger. But the subjects were rats, and ginger was taken internally rather than topically.

Make a ginger compress or paste by boiling water with 1 tablespoon of grated fresh gingerroot. Soak a washcloth in the mixture. When cool, apply the washcloth to the area where you're experiencing pain at least once per day for 15 to 30 minutes. Skin irritation is possible, so it's best to do a test on a small patch of skin first.

Take ginger internally by boiling water and steeping 2 teaspoons of gingerroot for 10 minutes. Enjoy 3 cups per day.

Interactions are possible. Let your doctor know first before you take large amounts of ginger.

Warm water with apple cider vinegar, lemon juice, and turmeric

Apple cider vinegar, lemon juice, and turmeric are each frequently recommended anecdotally for gout. Together, they make a pleasant beverage and remedy.

No strong research supports apple cider vinegar for gout, though studies show it may support the kidneys. Otherwise, research is promising for lemon juice and turmeric for lowering uric acid.

Mix juice from one squeezed half lemon into warm water. Combine with 2 teaspoons turmeric and 1 teaspoon apple cider vinegar. Adjust to taste. Drink two to three times per day.

Celery or celery seeds

Celery is a food traditionally used to treat urinary issues. For gout, extract and seeds of the vegetable have become popular home remedies.

Experimental use is well-documented, though scientific research is scant. It's thought that celery may reduce inflammation.

Adequate celery amounts for treating gout aren't documented. Try eating celery many times per day, especially raw celery sticks, juice, extract, or seeds.

If purchasing an extract or supplement, follow label directions closely.

Nettle tea

Stinging nettle (Urtica dioica) is an herbal remedy for gout that may reduce inflammation and pain.

Traditional use is frequently referred to in studies. There's still no research directly proving it works. One study showed it protected the kidneys, but the subjects were male rabbits, and kidney injury was induced by administration of gentamicin, an antibiotic.

To try this tea, brew a cup by boiling water. Steep 1 to 2 teaspoons of dried nettle per cup of water. Drink up to 3 cups per day.

Dandelion

Dandelion teas, extracts, and supplements are used to improve liver and kidney health.

They may lower uric acid levels in those at risk for kidney injury, as shown in a 2013 study and a 2016 study, but these were on rats. Dandelion is unproven to help gout.

You can use dandelion tea, an extract, or a supplement. Follow label directions closely.

Milk thistle seeds

Milk thistle is an herb used for liver health.

A 2016 study suggested it may lower uric acid in the midst of conditions that can hurt the kidneys, and another from 2013 supports it. However, both studies were on rats.

Follow dosing directions on a milk thistle supplement carefully or discuss it with your doctor.

Hibiscus

Hibiscus is a garden flower, food, tea, and traditional herbal remedy.

It may be a folk remedy used to treat gout. One study showed that hibiscus might lower uric acid levels, though this study was performed on rats.

Use a supplement, tea, or extract. Follow label directions closely.

Topical cold or hot application

Applying cold or hot water to inflamed joints may also be effective.

Studies and opinions on this are mixed. Soaking in cold water is most often recommended and considered most effective. Ice packs may also work.

Soaking in hot water is typically only recommended when inflammation isn't as intense.

Alternating hot and cold applications may also be helpful.

Apples

Natural health sites may recommend apples as part of gout-reducing diets. The claim: Apples contain malic acid, which lowers uric acid.

However, there aren't any studies supporting this for gout. Apples also contain fructose, which may trigger hyperuricemia, leading to gout flare-ups.

Eating one apple per day is good for overall health. It may be mildly beneficial for gout, but only if it doesn't add to excessive daily sugar consumption.

Bananas

Bananas are thought to be good for gout. They're potassium-rich, which helps the tissue and organs in the body to function properly.

Bananas also contain sugars, including fructose, which can be a gout trigger. Many foods are higher in potassium and lower in sugar than bananas, such as dark leafy greens and avocados.

Eat one banana per day for benefit. No studies yet support any benefit from bananas for gout.

Drinking plenty of water

A person with gout can reduce swelling by drinking plenty of water.

When a person has gout, they can experience significant swelling and inflammation. One of the ways to reduce swelling is by drinking more water.

Increasing fluid consumption can kick-start a person's kidneys to release excess fluid, which can reduce swelling in a person with gout.

Water is best, but other clear fluids, such as broths and herbal teas are also good choices. People should avoid alcohol and sodas, which are high in purines.

However, anyone with congestive heart failure or kidney disease should talk to their doctor before increasing their fluid intake.

Reducing stress

Heightened stress can worsen a person's gout symptoms. While it is not always possible to eliminate all sources of stress, the following tips might help:

- exercising, such as taking a brief walk, if the pain does not limit movement
- asking for time off from work
- journaling or reading a favorite book
- listening to music
- meditating

Getting enough rest can also help a person feel less stressed.

Increasing your fish intake

Fish contain anti-inflammatory compounds that help to enhance health overall. Some research has found some fish especially helpful in reducing uric acid levels.

Authors of a 2016 study found that taking tuna extract helped to reduce participants' serum uric acid levels. However, the participants did not have gout, so more research is necessary to confirm these results.

However, some nutrition websites list tuna as a high-purine food, so some people may find eating tuna worsens their symptoms.

In addition, the Arthritis Foundation list a number of other fish that contain high levels of purines, including anchovies, sardines, and cod.

Drinking coffee

Some people think drinking coffee may decrease the risk of experiencing gout.

A 2016 review and meta-analysis showed that those who drank more coffee were less likely to have gout. This may be because coffee can lower uric acid levels.

However, just because the study showed a correlation between higher coffee consumption and lower risk of gout, this does not mean that coffee caused the lower risk.

Drinking lemon water

The authors of a 2015 study found that adding the juice of two freshly squeezed lemons to 2 liters of water each day reduced uric acid in people with gout.

The researchers concluded that lemon water helps to neutralize uric acid in the body, thus helping to reduce levels.

Limiting alcohol intake

According to the Arthritis Foundation, drinking more than two liquor drinks or two beers per day increases a person's risk for gout.

Beer is high in purines, so avoiding it can benefit a person with gout.

Avoid sugary drinks

The heavy consumption of sugary drinks - such as sodas and sweetened juices - correlates with an increased risk of developing gout.

Sweetened drinks also add unnecessary calories to the diet, potentially causing weight gain and metabolic issues.

Avoiding high-purine meats

Some meats also contain high amounts of purines. Avoiding meats that contain high levels of purine might help to reduce a person's gout symptoms.

Meats and fish that are high in purines include:

- bacon
- turkey
- veal
- venison
- organ meats, such as liver
- anchovies
- sardines
- mussels
- herring
- cod
- haddock
- trout
- scallops

Epsom salts

Some people recommend a bath of Epsom salts to prevent gout attacks.

The idea is that Epsom salts are rich in magnesium, which may lower gout risk. However, studies show magnesium can't be adequately absorbed through skin to confer any health benefits.

To give Epsom salts a try, mix 1 to 2 cups in your bath. Soak your entire body or only specific joints for symptom relief.

Applying ice to affected joints

Applying a cloth-covered ice pack to the joint can help reduce gout-related inflammation.

Try applying an ice pack wrapped in a thin towel for 10 - 15 minutes at a time to help relieve pain.

If gout is affecting the feet, a person can also use a pack of frozen vegetables covered with a washcloth, as this may drape more easily over the feet.

Eat more low-purine foods

By switching from foods with a high purine content to those with a lower purine content, some people may be able to steadily lower their uric acid levels or at least avoid further increases. Some foods with low purine content include:

- low-fat and fat-free dairy products
- peanut butter and most nuts
- most fruits and vegetables
- coffee
- whole-grain rice, bread, and potatoes

Dietary changes alone will not get rid of gout, but they may help prevent flare-ups. It is also important to note that not everyone who gets gout eats a high-purine diet.

Other factors, such as genetic susceptibility, also play a role. African Americans are more vulnerable than white people to gout. Postmenopausal women and people with obesity also have a higher risk.

Avoid drugs that raise uric acid levels

Certain medications may elevate uric acid levels. These medicines include:

- diuretic drugs, such as furosemide (Lasix) and hydrochlorothiazide
- drugs that suppress the immune system, especially before or after an organ transplant
- low-dose aspirin

Drugs that raise uric acid levels may offer essential health benefits, however, so people should speak to a doctor before changing any medications.

Maintain a healthy body weight

Maintaining a healthy body weight may lower the risk of gout flares and heart disease.

Reaching a healthy body weight may help reduce the risk of gout flares. Obesity increases the risk of gout, especially in people of a younger age.

Being overweight also increases a person's risk of metabolic syndrome. It can raise blood pressure and cholesterol while increasing the risk of heart disease. While these effects are harmful in their own right, being overweight also has an association with a higher risk of elevated blood uric acid levels, raising the risk of gout.

Rapid weight loss, especially when it occurs due to fasting, may raise uric acid levels. Therefore, people should focus on making long-term sustainable changes to manage their weight, such as becoming more active, eating a balanced diet, and choosing nutrient-dense foods.

A GOUT-FRIENDLY MENU FOR ONE WEEK

Eating a gout-friendly diet will help you relieve the pain and swelling, while preventing future attacks.

Here is a sample gout-friendly menu for one week.

Monday

- **Breakfast:** Oats with Greek yogurt and 1/4 cup (about 31 grams) berries.
- **Lunch:** Quinoa salad with boiled eggs and fresh veggies.
- **Dinner:** Whole wheat pasta with roasted chicken, spinach, bell peppers and low-fat feta cheese.

Tuesday

- **Breakfast:** Smoothie with 1/2 cup (74 grams) blueberries, 1/2 cup (15 grams) spinach, 1/4 cup (59 ml) Greek yogurt and 1/4 cup (59 ml) low-fat milk.
- **Lunch:** Whole grain sandwich with eggs and salad.
- **Dinner:** Stir-fried chicken and vegetables with brown rice.

Wednesday

- **Breakfast:** Overnight oats — 1/3 cup (27 grams) rolled oats, 1/4 cup (59 ml) Greek yogurt, 1/3 cup (79 ml) low-fat milk, 1 tbsp (14 grams) chia seeds, 1/4 cup (about 31 grams) berries and 1/4 tsp (1.2 ml) vanilla extract. Let sit overnight.
- **Lunch:** Chickpeas and fresh vegetables in a whole wheat wrap.
- **Dinner:** Herb-baked salmon with asparagus and cherry tomatoes.

Thursday

- **Breakfast:** Overnight chia seed pudding — 2 tbsp (28 grams) chia seeds, 1 cup (240 ml) Greek yogurt and 1/2 tsp (2.5 ml) vanilla extract with sliced fruits of your choice. Let sit in a bowl or mason jar overnight.
- **Lunch:** Leftover salmon with salad.
- **Dinner:** Quinoa, spinach, eggplant and feta salad.

Friday

- **Breakfast:** French toast with strawberries.
- **Lunch:** Whole grain sandwich with boiled eggs and salad.
- **Dinner:** Stir-fried tofu and vegetables with brown rice.

Saturday

- **Breakfast:** Mushroom and zucchini frittata.
- **Lunch:** Leftover stir-fried tofu and brown rice.
- **Dinner:** Homemade chicken burgers with a fresh salad.

Sunday

- **Breakfast:** Two - egg omelet with spinach and mushrooms.
- **Lunch:** Chickpeas and fresh vegetables in a whole wheat wrap.
- **Dinner:** Scrambled egg tacos - scrambled eggs with spinach and bell peppers on whole wheat tortillas.

OTHER TIPS FOR REDUCING GOUT FLARE-UPS

Eliminate diet triggers

Diet is often closely related to gout flareups and pain. Avoiding triggers and keeping to a good gout diet is an important remedy in and of itself.

Studies show red meat, seafood, sugar, and alcohol are the most likely triggers. Stick to low-sugar fruits, vegetables, whole grains, nuts, legumes, and low-fat dairy instead.

Hydrate often

Drinking plenty of water is important to kidney function. Keeping the kidneys in good shape can also reduce uric acid crystal buildup and gout attacks.

Make sure to stay hydrated and drink plenty of water, which can be helpful for gout. No studies show it can replace gout treatments, however.

Get plenty of rest

Gout attacks can interfere with movement and mobility.

To avoid worsening symptoms, relax and stay put while joints are inflamed. Avoid exercising, bearing heavy weights, and using joints excessively, which can worsen the pain and duration of a flare-up.

THE GOUT DIET

Gout, also known as gouty arthritis is caused by the buildup of uric acid, a metabolite of protein and can be extremely painful. Gout generally occurs more often in men and second most in post menopausal women.

The excess of uric acid leads to the formation of small crystals of urate (uric acid crystals). Some of these crystal deposits form in the synovial fluid (lubricating fluid around joints) that then cause inflammation and result in this painful condition.

When someone has a gout attack it can be extremely painful in the area of the big toe and signs also include redness and swelling in the joint. Other joints may be affected and the pain can be so intense that even touching the area can be excruciating.

Causes of gout include: a diet high in hydrogenated fats, alcohol, conventional meat and refined carbohydrates. Also having conditions such as insulin resistance, obesity, kidney disease, stress, high blood pressure, and an acidic system can greatly increase the risk of developing gout.

If you want to overcome gout then diet is key. Follow this gout diet for fast relief and do actually address the cause of gout and get rid of it forever.

- **High-fiber foods** – High fiber foods include fruits, vegetables, nuts and seeds that are high in fiber which can help reduce uric acid.
- **Potassium-rich foods** – Foods high in potassium like avocado, raw cultured dairy, coconut water, salmon, squash, bananas and apricots can help balance intracellular fluid relieving gout.
- **Fresh berries and cherries** – Berries and especially cherries can help neutralize uric acid.
- **Wild-caught fish** – Omega-3s help reduce inflammation and can help overcome gout pain.
- **Water** – Drink plenty of water, at least 8 oz every 2 hours to flush uric acid out of your system.

You also want to avoid the following foods:

- **Foods high in purines** – Purines are an amino acid that forms uric acid. Foods that have purines include: fatty red meat, shellfish, small fish, mushrooms, organ meats, peas, lentils, and spinach.
- **Fried foods and hydrogenated oils** – Fried foods and hydrogenated oils like soybean, vegetable, corn, and canola oil can aggravate gout.
- **Sodium** – A diet high in sodium can cause tissue swelling and increase gout symptoms.
- **Alcohol** – Increases uric acid and toxicity of the liver.
- **Refined carbohydrates** – Sugar and other refined carbohydrates can make insulin resistance and gout worse.

THE BOTTOM LINE

Plenty of options are available for helping or preventing gout attacks at home. Most are natural and have little to no side effects.

Always check with your doctor first before adding a supplement to your regimen. Interactions and side effects could be possible with herbal supplements.

Never replace your established, prescribed gout treatments with a home remedy without informing your doctor. None of the herbal supplements recommended are regulated by the U.S. Food and Drug Administration for what they contain or how well they work. Only purchase supplements from trusted companies for safety.

If your gout pain is considerable, sudden, or intense - or if home remedies cease to work - contact your doctor immediately.

CONCLUSION

Thank you for purchasing this book. I know there are many books on *Gout Natural Treatment and Prevention* out there, but you chose this one. I'm incredibly grateful to you, grateful for taking a chance on this read. And I sincerely wish you the best on all your adventures of KILLING GOUT!

If you know of anyone else who may benefit from the useful tips and guides for *BEATING GOUT* that are revealed in this book, please help me inform them of this book. I would greatly appreciate it.

Finally, if you enjoyed this book and feel that this book has been beneficial to you, please take a couple of minutes to share your thoughts and post a REVIEW on Amazon. Your feedback will help me to continue to write other books on diseases treatment topic that helps you get the best results. Furthermore, if you write a simple REVIEW with positive words for this book on Amazon, you can help hundreds or perhaps thousands of other readers who may want to save their life from stroke. Like you, they worked hard for every penny they spend on books. With the information and recommendation you provide, they would be more likely to take action right away. We really look forward to reading your review.

From the bottom of my heart, I thank you so much for staying with us during this book and for reading it through to the end. We really hope that you have enjoyed the contents!

Thanks again for your support and good luck!

If you enjoy my book, please write a POSITIVE REVIEW on Amazon.

-- Dr. Edward Thomas --

CHECK OUT OTHER BOOKS

Go here to check out other related books that might interest you:

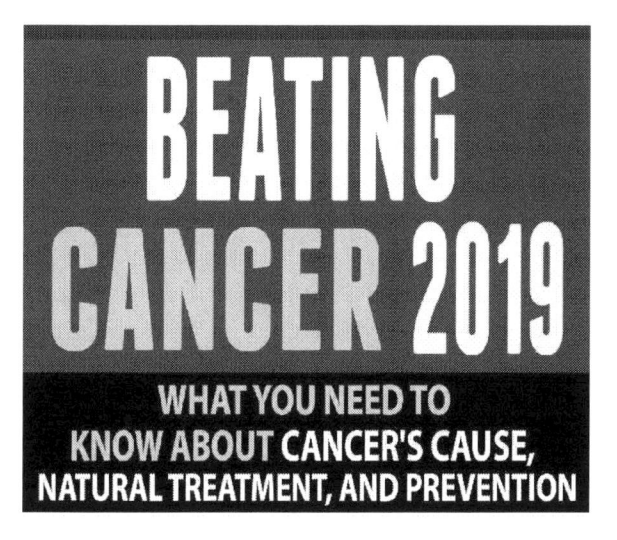

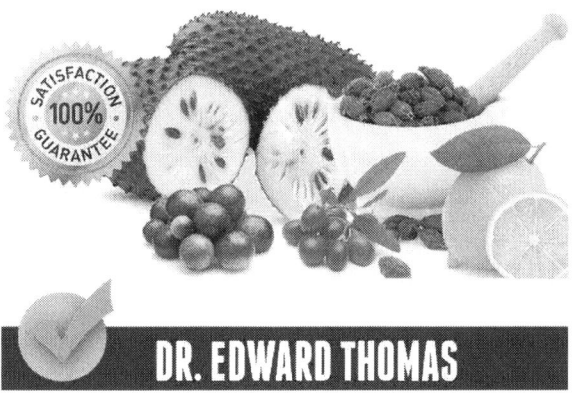

BEATING CANCER 2019: What You Need To Know About Cancer's Cause, Natural Treatment, And Prevention!

https://www.amazon.com/dp/B07R6MZ4VH

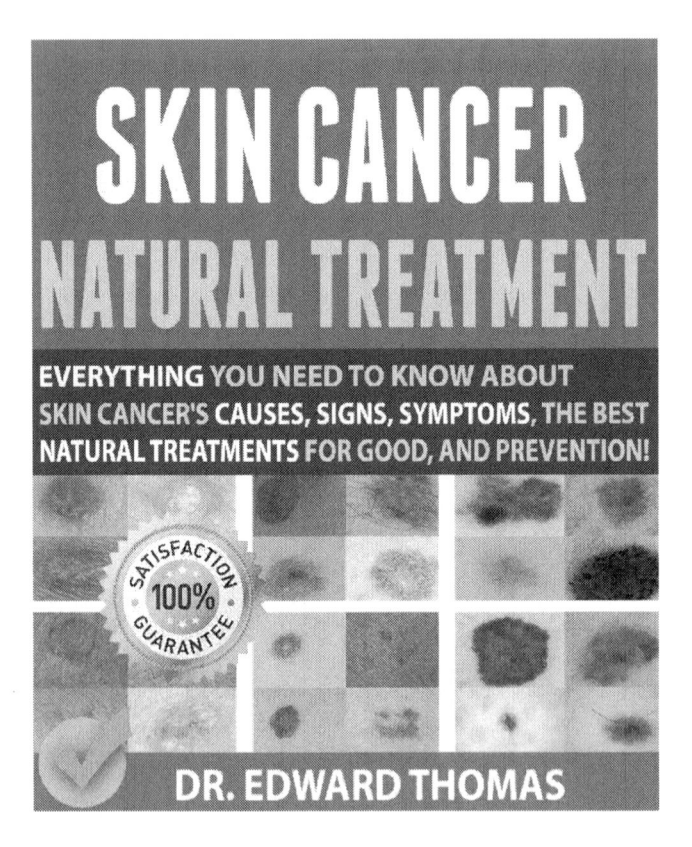

Stroke Natural Treatment: Everything You Need To Know About Stroke's Causes, Signs, Symptoms, The Best Natural Treatments For Good, And Prevention!

https://www.amazon.com/dp/B07XB2B9SP

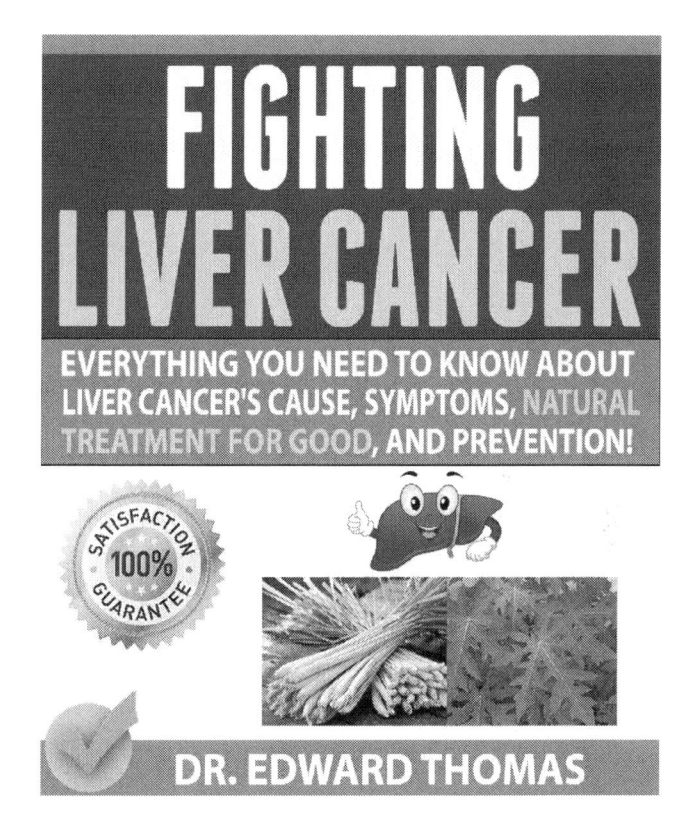

FIGHTING LIVER CANCER: Everything You Need To Know About Liver Cancer's Cause, Symptoms, The Best Natural Treatment For Good, And Prevention!

https://www.amazon.com/dp/B07SCQMS3K

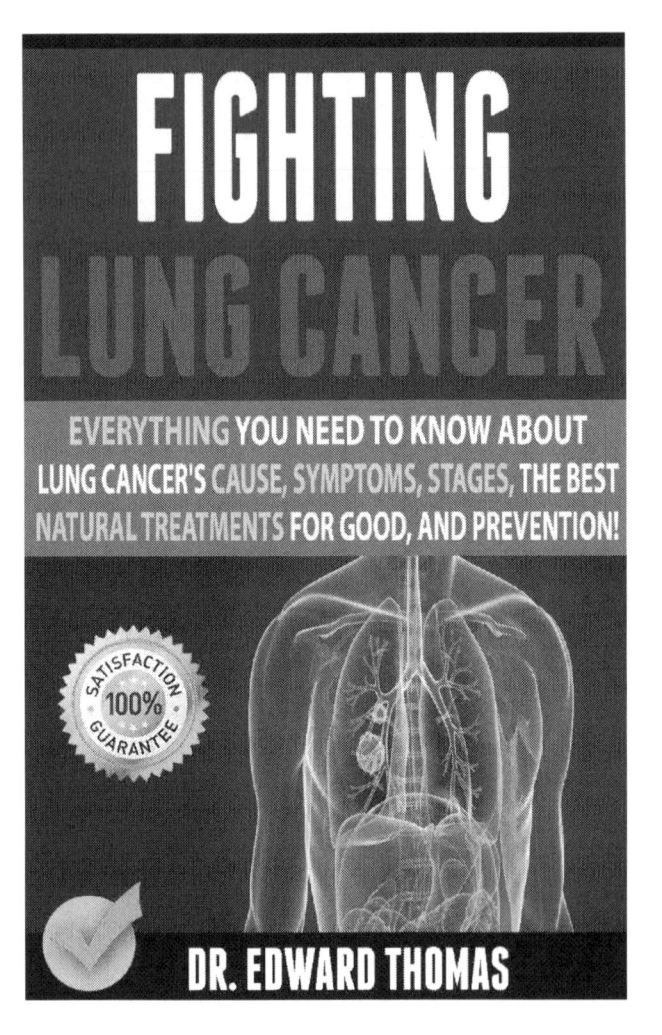

Fighting Lung Cancer: Everything You Need To Know About Lung Cancer's Cause, Symptoms, Stages, The Best Natural Treatments For Good, And Prevention!

https://www.amazon.com/dp/B07XB8H9G5

Best Cancer-Fighting Foods: Over 35+ Super Foods To Reduce Cancer Risk, Fight Cancer, Boost Your Energy, And Restore Your Health

https://www.amazon.com/dp/B07WHS5JF2

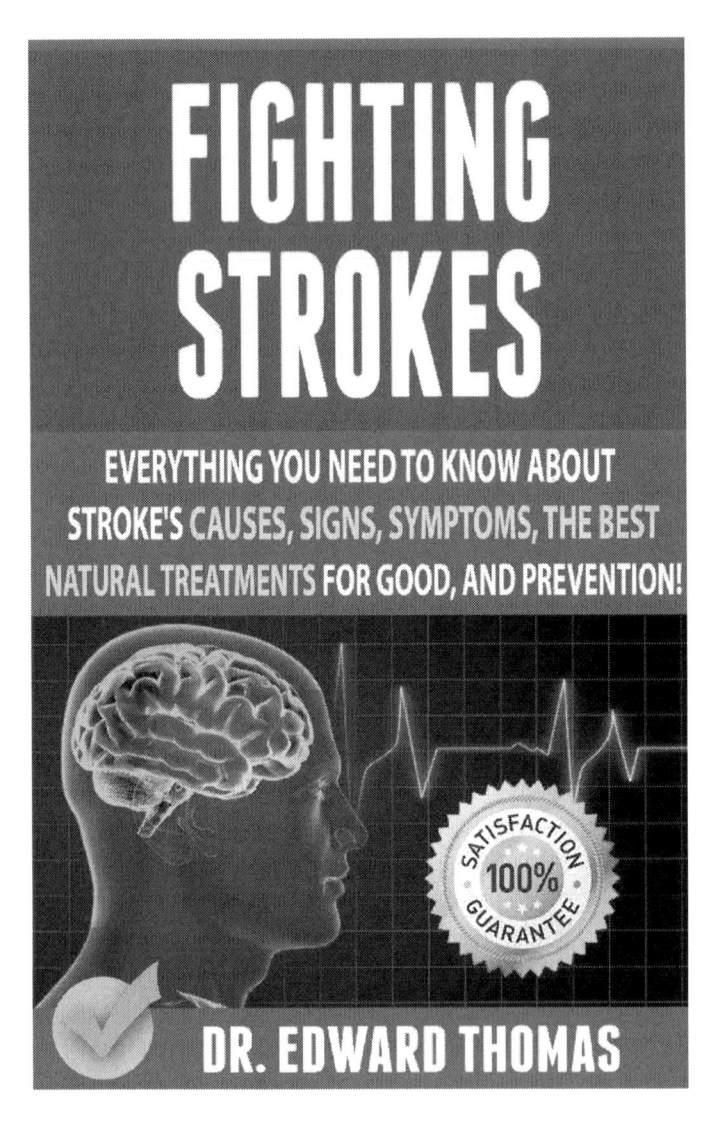

Fighting Stroke: Everything You Need To Know About Stroke's Causes, Signs, Symptoms, The Best Natural Treatments For Good, And Prevention!

https://www.amazon.com/dp/B081NJ2MSB

HOW TO GET PREGNANT FAST & NATURALLY

THE COMPLETE GUIDE, TIPS & HACKS TO GETTING PREGNANT EASILY, QUICKLY AND NATURALLY

JOEY BERRY

How To Get Pregnant Fast & Naturally: The Complete Guide, Tips & Hacks To Getting Pregnant Easily, Quickly And Naturally

https://www.amazon.com/dp/B07WJJYQZ4

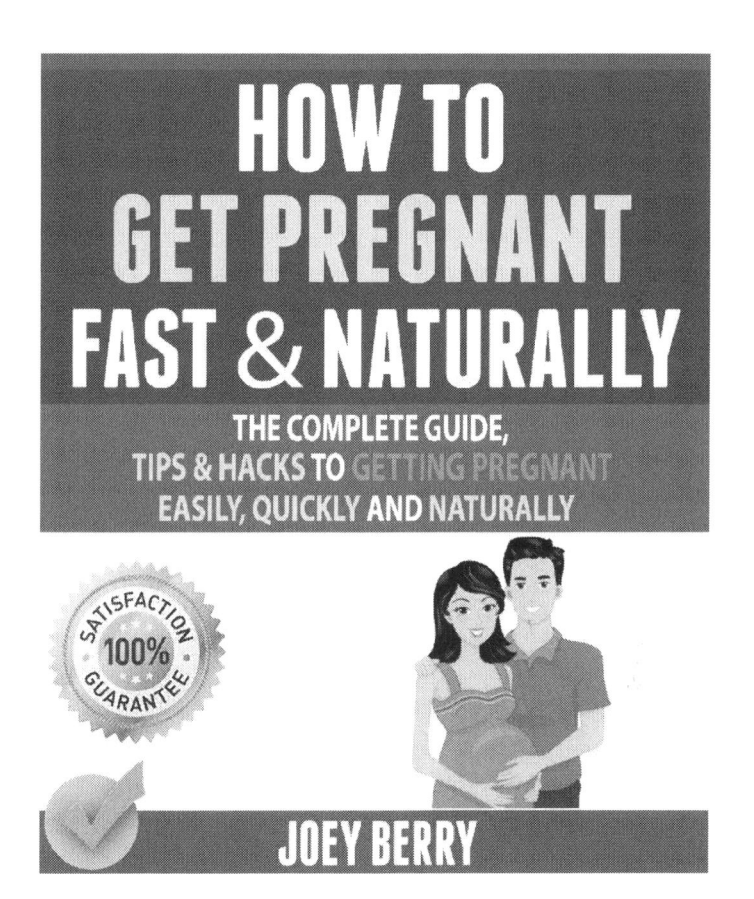

Made in the USA
Coppell, TX
02 October 2020